Self-determined Dying
Manual for a rational Suicide

The Method "Carotid Artery"

Self-determined Dying
Manual for a rational Suicide
The Method "Carotid Artery"

First published April 2020

Jessica Düber
Orleansstraße 22
31135 Hildesheim

Printversion by
Amazon Media EU S.à r.l., 5 Rue Plaetis,
L-2338 Luxembourg

ISBN 9798636838548

Foreword

On 26.02.2020, the Federal Constitutional Court declared the controversial paragraph 217 of the German Penal Code null and void. The right to self-determination with regard to decisions concerning one's own death was thus confirmed. The decision states that the right to self-determined death includes the freedom to commit suicide. It explicitly states that this right to self-determination is due to every person - even in the absence of illness. In order to put this right into practice, professional help must now be available to people. Of course, such assistance must be based on certain rules and criteria of due diligence that allow for a responsible implementation of the judgement. Exactly what implementation will look like now will become clear in the coming months. I believe, however, that this positive development should not lead us to rely exclusively on the ideas of the Members of the Bundestag. Despite the positive verdict in February, it seems to me to be a good idea to continue to familiarise ourselves personally with the possibilities of rational suicide. Autonomous possibilities for action always mean an increase in personal freedom.

Recently, I have received more frequent inquiries concerning the correct implementation of a suicide by compression of the carotid arteries (arteria carotis).

While looking through the available literature on this method, I came across quite comprehensive explanations as well as instructions that propagate the method without going into the underlying pathophysiological aspects and the resulting needs for practical implementation. For some people this may be enough - I would like to express this without criticism, because it is very important to me not to complicate methods for rational suicide by unnecessary theoretical explanations. However, I believe that more comprehensive information on the basics and practical implementation is needed to seriously address the question of whether interrupting the oxygen supply by compressing the carotid arteries is a suitable method for a painless and peaceful, self-determined death. The following paper should therefore provide an opportunity for interested readers to gain an overview of the method "Carotid Artery", as I would like to call it here.

When I wrote my first book on the subject of self-determined dying in 2017, I did not include the method "Carotid Artery". At that time I was interested in including possibilities for which there was already a minimum amount of empirical data. In the meantime, the conditions under which I would like to present methods for self-determined dying and bring them into public discussion have changed. I am not exclusively interested in ready-made recommendations, but in pointing out options and a possible resulting discussion or even optimizations of these options. In my opinion, there are still some open questions and aspects of the compression method that need closer examination. So if you are interested in dealing with the advantages and disadvantages of a method on a theoretical basis, this paper may be of benefit to you. If you are looking for a quick guide that describes and recommends a method without further hesitation, this paper might not be right for you.

A great advantage of the method is that it offers the possibility of dying in a self-determined way without the need to purchase the necessary materials. With methods that use drug combinations or inert gases, it is always a prerequisite that the utensils have either already been procured beforehand or that there are still procurement options available in the case of a wish to die. One could therefore regard the carotid artery - method as a kind of "emergency plan" and familiarise oneself with it in order to have an alternative for a self-determined dying in a case in which other methods are no longer feasible. All in all, I see the need to examine methods for rational suicide that can be carried out without having to rely on aids to which access can be restricted. The "Helium" and "Chloroquine" methods I presented in the 2017 handbook and also in updated versions of 2019 are now good and proven methods - however, it is possible that access to pure helium and also to chloroquine will be restricted by government regulations in the future and we should be prepared to be able to keep our self-determination at the end of life independent of external supply sources.

Basic principles of the method

The head arteries run along both sides of the neck. They are called carotid arteries (arteria carotis communis). The carotid artery (arteria carotis communis) divides into an inner (arteria carotis interna) and an outer (arteria carotis externa) carotid artery on both the right and left side of the neck (approximately at the level of the 4th cervical vertebra). Since this division runs like a fork, the branching point is also called the carotid bifurcation (bifurcatio carotidis).

Through the carotid arteries, the head and neck area is supplied with blood and thus with oxygen. The brain with all its vital functions is therefore dependent on a supply through the carotid arteries (the respective inner carotid artery is "responsible" for the arterial flow to the brain).

This fact is used in suicide by squeezing the carotid artery and thus stopping the flow of oxygen-rich arterial blood to the brain. Without oxygen, the brain dies. Since the brain is responsible for controlling breathing, breathing stops as a result of brain death. If the heart is no longer supplied with oxygen by breathing, there is also cardiac arrest. Since the method is carried out with the aid of a ligature system (for example, a tension belt or tourniquet), the oxygen supply to the brain remains permanently interrupted even after unconsciousness sets in. The rapid onset of unconsciousness is then followed by death. According to Docker, unconsciousness occurs within one minute; death occurs within a few minutes (see Docker, Chris, 2015: Five Last Acts - The Exit Path. p. 209).

There is another mechanism in this method of suicide that can lead to death. An occurrence is not very likely, but possible - so I will briefly describe the mechanism. It is important to note that it is, so to speak, an effect whose occurrence means a quick death and which would therefore be "welcome" - but when the carotid arteries are squeezed, one does not try to trigger the reflex described below. The suicide method "carotid artery" is based exclusively on cutting off the oxygen supply to the brain. Nevertheless:

Directly above the branching of the carotid artery known as the carotid bifurcation lies the sinus caroticus (carotissinus). This is a small thickening or dilatation at the very beginning of the internal carotid artery (the dilatation is located directly after the branch). The vascular walls of the carotid sinus have pressure receptors (pressor receptors or baroreceptors) that react to a change in arterial blood pressure. By increasing the pressure, the body's protective mechanism, a reflex slowing of the heart rate and a reduction in blood pressure occurs. This reaction can also be triggered by strong external pressure on the carotid bifurcation (carotid sinus reflex). This can lead to a significant drop in blood pressure; under certain circumstances, triggering the carotid sinus reflex can also lead to cardiac arrest with fatal consequences.

No compression of the airways!

The basic functioning of the methodology has already been explained above. For a better understanding, some explanations follow.

It seems important to me at first to make it clear that the method has nothing to do with "suffocation". Of course, death is caused by a lack of oxygen in the brain, but the compression of the throat should not involve squeezing the windpipe. Compression is performed in the upper part of the neck (far above the Adam's apple, almost directly under the chin). Free breathing is therefore not hindered by this method.

For a long time the pathophysiology of strangulation was not known and I assume that in some people an intuitive dislike of this method is also based on a certain ignorance of the exact mechanisms. Throughout the centuries, there have been various models for explaining death by strangulation; one assumption that is still widely accepted today as the cause of death, particularly in the case of hanging, was that death occurs by broken neck. This assumption is now obsolete; only a fall from a great height can lead to a broken neck when using the hanging method. Likewise, the assumption that death occurs by compression of the respiratory tract has only been disproved over time (see Swiss Society of Forensic Medicine, 2012: Damage by Strangulation. p. 5ff). However, the general idea that the respiratory tract is compressed during strangulation still holds true. In criminal law contexts this may occur frequently (also due to the fact that the generation of additional suffering may be intentional), but in our objective it is completely unnecessary. Airway compression also requires a much greater force than is necessary to compress the carotid arteries.

The pros of the method "Carotid Artery"

Even if the method "Carotid Artery" should not be the method of first choice for you, I still think it is useful to be familiar with the procedure. There may be situations in which the use of another method is not possible because you do not (or no longer) have the necessary privacy. This would be the case, for example, if self-determined dying can no longer be carried out at home as planned, but you are already in a hospital or other care facility due to an incident. It would also be conceivable that one still has the necessary privacy, but has failed to obtain all the necessary utensils for the preferred method (for example a helium cylinder, a pressure reducer etc. or certain combinations of medication) beforehand. Under changed circumstances, procurement may prove difficult; the availability of required materials may also have been further restricted by the government. So let us assume that you are in a situation where your "method of first choice" is not feasible. What would you do? I have to admit that I was very impressed by the question posed by Chris Docker in the introduction to the compression method in his book - he writes there that he likes to ask the participants of his workshops at the beginning if they would know how they could do it if they came to the conclusion that they wanted to end their lives NOW. They should imagine that they only had half an hour to get the materials they needed. Would you have enough knowledge of a method to die self-determinedly within half an hour without any preparation? Docker expresses the wish that after reading through his chapter "Compression" (possibly several times) every person should be able to answer this question positively (see Docker, Chris, 2015: Five Last Acts - The Exit Path. p. 211).

I see it similarly - so let's look at the method of eventually having more options - an increase in alternatives can mean a gain in personal freedom. With regard to the little preparation work and the few required, always accessible, cheap (or free) and in its availability not regulable materials, the method is certainly very advantageous.

Detailed description of the functionality

The following pathophysiological mechanisms may underlie the damage or death caused by compression of the neck:

- Compression of the blood vessels - here a distinction is made between obstruction of the carotid arteries, the jugular veins and the vertebral arteries. For an obstruction of the carotid arteries a necessary weight of about 5kg is assumed, for an obstruction of the jugular veins a weight of 2kg and for an obstruction of the vertebral arteries 15-30kg

- Compression of the airways - the required force is at least 8-12kg

- Cardiac arrest through the so-called carotid sinus reflex. This is a reflex response to pressure exerted on the pressor receptors of the carotid sinus

For us and our planned procedure only the compression of the blood vessels described in the first paragraph is interesting or desirable. A cardiac arrest by triggering the carotid sinus reflex is rare, but possible. Whether a carotid sinus reflex is triggered depends very much on the overall health of a person. In particular, older men with pre-existing conditions such as coronary heart disease, hypertension and diabetes mellitus may have a hypersensitive carotissinus, a condition in which (in simple terms) the baroreceptors are more sensitive. The fact that one does not know exactly how sensitive one's own carotid sinus is to pressure is actually mainly relevant when the compression method is practiced in advance. Here, care should be taken not to apply very high pressure in practice situations. The point of training is to get a practical idea of the procedure - it is not about exerting so much pressure that stimulation of the carotid sinus occurs or that clouding of consciousness already occurs.

We now want to take a closer look at the actual implementation. In the following I will describe two methods of compression - firstly, compression using a tourniquet and secondly, compression using a ratchet strap. These two methods are also presented by Docker (see Docker, Chris, 2015: Five Last Acts - The Exit Path. p. 209-275). In Germany, the use of cable ties seems to have gained a certain popularity after Peter Puppe introduced the method using cable ties - but without going into the pathophysiological mechanisms and the resulting peculiarities that should be taken into account in the practical implementation (see Puppe, Peter, 2017: Gentle Euthanasia without Doctor. p. 41ff.). I will not go into detail about the use of cable ties - of course cable ties can be used, but in my opinion there are more suitable materials for a compression of the neck. But this is possibly also a question of taste. I also do not go into the possibility of hanging.

Besides the use of a tourniquet and a ratchet strap, Docker also describes the technique that achieves compression by wrapping the strap around several times - I will not describe this possibility here either. For a comprehensive introduction to the topic, I suggest you anyway to at least read through Docker's book - there you will also find interesting literature references for a deeper understanding of many aspects. In addition - even if you don't know the English language very well - it might be very helpful to have a look at the many drawings and illustrations Docker has included.

The tourniquet method works on the principle of shortening a band by rotation. Basically you only need a ribbon to tie the neck and a stick or rod to shorten the ribbon by rotation.

Suppose you want to use a necktie as your ribbon. This must be knotted beforehand, because we need a band that is closed all around (a "loop"). Of course it is easier to knot the band before you put it around your neck, because it is important to use a knot that is really tight. There are types of knots that can easily come loose again when you pull on them - but there are also knots that get tighter and tighter the more you pull on them. A knot that is really easy to tie is the reef knot (also called square knot). Docker recommends its use in his book and also points out that a reef knot can turn into a granny' knot when tied the wrong way, which is much less durable (see Docker, Chris, 2015: Five Last Acts - The Exit Path. p. 215).

Another knot that is quite safe would be the so-called zeppelin bend also called rosendahl bend). You might want to take a look at the knotting possibilities in advance - but I think the reef knot is the knot that many of us can tie intuitively as a so-called "double knot". To be on the safe side, it would be possible to make several of these knots in a row to prevent them from opening.

The resulting loop should only be wide enough so that it can just be pulled over the head - not bigger. If you want to make the knot only after you have already wrapped the ribbon around your neck, you should knot the ribbon in such a way that you can slide about four fingers between neck and ribbon (so there should be about 5-7cm free between neck and ribbon). A rod is then inserted into this gap between neck and band. Many things are suitable as a stick - for example a wooden cooking spoon, a long artist's brush or a long cosmetic brush. Large sticks can also be used (for example a walking stick or a crutch). When the stick is turned (either forward or backward, it doesn't matter), the strap is shortened and thus becomes tighter. If you lose consciousness and let go of the pole, it will prevent the band from opening again by resting (depending on the direction of rotation and length chosen beforehand) either on the shoulder blades or on the chest. The method works both in a sitting and lying position. If the person is lying down, the rod would come to rest (depending on the direction of rotation) either on the chest or at the back on the floor, mattress or similar.

A lot can be taken as a band. For example, Docker recommends so-called "Rufflette", a strong fabric tape made of pure cotton that is used to sew curtains (see Docker, Chris, 2015: Five Last Acts - The Exit Path. p. 218ff.). However, he also reports on cases where nylon tights have been successfully used and pleads for being creative with the materials. However, one should make sure that the fabric is tear-resistant. An elastic material that is only elastic up to a certain degree and then no longer stretchable but stable is also a possibility. Yoga straps and lashing straps for luggage could also be used. The ratchet straps described below can also be used for the Tourniquet method (you only have to cut off the end where the ratchet is (see Docker, Chris, 2015: Five Last Acts - The Exit Path. p. 218ff.). If you notice during previous exercises that the chosen material cuts unpleasantly into the skin, it is possible to put something underneath as padding. Here too, basically anything can be used. Very practical, however, are headbands - for example made of soft fleece (see Docker, Chris, 2015: Five Last Acts - The Exit Path. p. 219-220).

Another possibility is to use a tension belt with a ratchet. If you have mastered the use of the ratchet, this is a very comfortable method of achieving neck compression. The strap fits snugly around the neck and no twisting cuts into the skin.

Before using a ratchet, make sure you are familiar with its handling. First read the operating instructions and practice lashing and unlatching the ratchet to an object. It is very unpleasant to have a ratchet around your neck when you cannot handle it and may not be able to loosen it.

A very important aspect, which is generally valid for all methods of strangulation, is the following: If the tightening of the strap, tension belt etc. is done too hesitantly and too slowly, a "swollen" feeling can occur in the head, the conscious experience of which can be unpleasant. The reason for this becomes clear if you look again at the forces necessary for the compression of the blood vessels, which are listed at the beginning of this chapter. For the compression of the carotid arteries about 5kg of force is needed, for the compression of the jugular veins only about 2kg. Now the carotid arteries are responsible for transporting fresh arterial blood to the brain, while the jugular veins transport the "used", low-oxygen blood back again. Now, if a hesitant and weak compression only compresses the veins, the blood that is still being transported through the arteries to the brain cannot flow out. It accumulates in the head. According to Docker, the fact that the blood cannot flow off and thus causes a disturbance of the blood circulation, eventually leads to no or less fresh blood flowing in through the carotid arteries, which at some point would have the same effect as the rapid and strong impression of the carotid arteries (see Docker, Chris, 2015: Five Last Acts - The Exit Path. pp. 212-213). Nevertheless, Docker points out several times that it is very important to apply compression quickly and powerfully at the same time; in this way, the carotid arteries are squeezed at the same time as the jugular veins and the arterial flow to the brain is stopped (see Docker, Chris, 2015: Five Last Acts - The Exit Path. p. 222). Unpleasant feelings can thus be avoided.

Survival of the brainstem?

Once again I would like to come to the necessary forces described at the beginning of the previous chapter, which must be applied to the blood vessels in order to block them.

I have listed there the forces needed for the obstruction of the carotid arteries and the jugular veins - the meaning of the different forces needed was also explained in the previous chapter. But what about the vertebral arteries also listed there, whose obstruction requires a force of about 15-30kg (i.e. a much higher force than is needed to obstruct the carotid arteries and the jugular veins)?

The vertebral arteries originate in the thoracic cavity and supply different areas with their branches. Via the arteria basilaris and with the influx from the circulus arteriosus willisii they are responsible for supplying the brain stem. The brain stem is responsible for controlling vital functions such as breathing, blood pressure and reflexes. Due to their course through the foramen transversarium (bone openings in the transverse process of the cervical vertebrae), the vertebral arteries are well protected and cannot be blocked by strangulation. An obstruction of the vertebral arteries would only be possible by applying a high force - but since the forces required to obstruct the airways are much lower, applying the necessary forces would also cause a blockage of the airways, which would not be desirable.

This fact therefore means that if the neck is compressed (as recommended, vigorously and courageously), there is usually only an obstruction of the jugular veins and carotid arteries. The brain stem continues to be supplied via the vertebral arteries. There has therefore been a debate in professional circles as to whether there is a risk of death of the cerebrum in the case of compression, but whether the brain stem can survive under certain circumstances. In simple terms, the cerebrum is responsible for cognitive functions such as thinking and acting. If the cerebrum dies during compression but the brain stem survives, the result would probably be survival in a purely vegetative state. Pieter Admiraal first stated in 2004 at a meeting of the NuTech group (New Technologies in Self - Deliverance; a loose association of scientists and other people committed to developing practical solutions for self-determined dying) that in his opinion it is possible that heart and respiratory functions can be maintained by the survival of the brain stem after using the compression method (see Chabot, Boudewijn, 2014: A Way to Die. p. 87 and Docker, Chris, 2015: Five Last Acts - The Exit Path. p. 230ff.). In his book "A Way to Die" from 2014, Boudewijn Chabot takes up this criticism and introduces the idea of possibly being able to avoid the risk of brain stem survival by pulling a plastic bag over the head in addition to the compression (see Chabot, Boudewijn, 2014: A Way to Die. p. 87, 89). I interpret it to mean that Chabot, in his book "Dignified Dying" of 2015 (which can be seen as the follow-up book to "A Way to Die" published in 2014, where the title was changed and the content revised and updated), has somewhat softened his criticism of the method. Although he still writes that there is a concern that the brain stem will continue to be supplied by the vertebral arteries, he states that it is likely that, despite continued supply by the vertebral arteries, the brain stem will also die - due to swelling and bleeding that occurs inside the brain because of the lack of blood supply through the carotid arteries (see Chabot, Boudewijn, 2015: Dignified Dying. p. 92).

Docker argues in a similar way. He describes that swelling and bleeding, which are associated with the death of the cerebrum, probably lead to the death of the brain stem, because the swelling and bleeding have no place to spread in the brain - except downwards into the area of the brain stem (see Docker, Chris, 2015: Five Last Acts - The Exit Path. p. 230, 232ff.). However, he also points out that the corresponding processes are complex and difficult to determine in a direct way - brain scans during self-determined dying by means of the compression method have not yet been carried out. Some cases are known in which persons survived after strangulation in a permanently vegetative state. However, Docker states that in all cases documented to date in which the compression method was performed with the aim of suicide, complete death rather than a permanent vegetative state occurred.

Further research is necessary to find out what the actual cause is here. The few cases documented to date in which a permanent vegetative state occurred instead of death, all occurred during *temporary* compression. These temporary compressions occurred, for example, when one person was strangled by another person, when the so-called stranglehold was used in police work or during the so-called "Choking Game" ("strangle game", "fainting game" or similar) - a game that is sometimes used in youth cultures, in which a temporary blockage of the arterial supply is intended to trigger a feeling of "euphoria" due to the resulting lack of oxygen (see Docker, Chris, 2015: Five Last Acts - The Exit Path. p. 230, 231). Docker cites as a major difference between temporary and permanent compression the fact that during permanent compression (as is ensured when using a tourniquet, ratchet strap or the like) any blood that may still be reaching the brain cannot drain off permanently, which means that the pressure there continues to rise. However, he also discusses other possible reasons for brain stem death - including disorders of brain metabolism or a lack of supply not only of oxygen but also of glucose and other nutrients. In this respect, he once again emphasizes that, in view of the complex processes involved, it is not yet possible to say with one hundred percent certainty which factors ultimately lead to the death of the brain stem after the cortex has died (see Docker, Chris, 2015: Five Last Acts - The Exit Path. p. 234, 235).

Additional use of a plastic bag?

Although Docker is of the opinion that the use of a plastic bag as additional protection is not absolutely necessary (see Docker, Chris, 2015: Five Last Acts - The Exit Path. p. 230, 232), he nevertheless presents the method. Due to the discussions about a possible survival of the brainstem resulting in a permanent vegetative state, possibilities were sought to make the method "Carotid Artery" safer. In the "Carotid Artery compression plus plastic bag" method, an additional plastic bag is pulled over the head. Docker describes that the easiest way is to place the bag at the neck under the compression strap (i.e. you would first place the bag over the head and then pull the compression strap over it; this way the bag at the neck does not need any additional fastening (e.g. an elastic band in the hem or similar). If the respiratory function were to be maintained by the brain stem, the oxygen in the bag would be used up after some time - then the lack of oxygen would also lead to a failure of the vegetative functions (see Docker, Chris, 2015: Five Last Acts - The Exit Path. p. 230, 238-239). Chabot also describes this way of using a plastic bag (see Chabot, Boudewijn, 2014: A Way to Die. p. 89). Chabot also writes that the increasing CO_2 content in the bag (which is not, as for example in the helium method, displaced from the bag) is not consciously experienced, because when the CO_2 content in the bag increases, one is already in a state of unconsciousness (see Chabot, Boudewijn, 2014: A Way to Die. p. 89). This would prevent unpleasant reactions to the increasing CO_2 content inside the bag. However, Chabot also writes that this method is still in an experimental phase and that no empirical data are available on its use yet - a general discussion would therefore be very desirable (see Chabot, Boudewijn, 2014: A Way to Die. p. 89).

Physical findings after death by strangulation

It may not be important for everyone what effects of an optical nature can occur after death by strangulation. Due to the differences in the forces acting and the overall process, the externally visible signs can also be very different. When compression is applied with an aid (tourniquet, tension belt with ratchet etc.), so-called ligature marks may occur. The extent of these ligature marks depends on the utensil used - in the case of narrow utensils (rope, cable ties, etc.) the occurrence of a furrow is probable, which is clearly defined and may be deeply cut into the skin. In the case of wider utensils, blurred marks usually occur, which are not incised so deeply into the skin. They can also be completely absent if wide and soft utensils were used (see Swiss Society of Forensic Medicine, 2012: Damage caused by strangulation. S. 8-9). Underlaying a cushion can also change the appearance of a strangulation mark.

A congestion syndrome can occur due to an obstruction in the venous blood flow caused by obstruction of the veins while the arterial inflow is still (even partially) intact. The consequence of a congestion syndrome can be the development of so-called petechiae. These are bleedings from the capillaries into the skin or into the mucous membranes (mainly into the facial skin, the conjunctiva of the eyes, the mucous membranes of the mouth, lips, nose, epiglottis and larynx, eardrums, tongue, throat, tonsils) (see Swiss Society of Forensic Medicine, 2012: Damage caused by strangulation. S. 10). According to Docker, the occurrence of cyanosis (blue coloration of skin and mucous membranes due to reduced oxygen saturation of the blood) is also possible (see Docker, Chris, 2015: Five Last Acts - The Exit Path. p. 253).

CPSIA information can be obtained
at www.ICGtesting.com
Printed in the USA
LVHW092058210322
714007LV00007B/951